Primer on Neurosteroids and Chronic Pain Care

Forest Tennant
DrPH, MPH, MD

American Dictionary
Primer: any small book of elementary principals

Published by
Arachnoiditis Hope
A project of the Tennant Foundation

ISBN: 9781955934541
Library of Congress Control Number: 2026917720

Special discounts are available on quantity purchases by corporations, associations, educators, and others. For details, contact one of the parties listed below.

Nancy Kriskovich Tel: (406)249-2002;
or email snkriskovich@gmail.com

Tennant Foundation
336-338 S. Glendora Ave.
West Covina, CA 91790-3043
Ph: 626-716-2689
Fax: 626-919-7497
Email: tennantfoundation92@gmail.com

PUBLICATION DEVELOPMENT

Rebecca Cholcher-Marino

Nancy Kriskovich

TABLE OF CONTENTS

AUTHORS NOTES

Neurosteroids are hormone substances that are synthesized in the brain and spinal cord (central nervous system). They have multiple functions in the CNS. Of relevance to this "Primer" they have potent healing and neuroregenerative properties. They also have innate ability to relieve pain and suppress inflammation. After many years of laboratory research and elementary clinical research, enough practical knowledge has been gained that neurosteroids now have a therapeutic role in chronic pain care. This primer provides guidance on the common chronic pain issues and how and where the neurosteroids fit in. Neurosteroids are easy to administer and remarkably safe for pain care problems.

INTRODUCTION

Neurosteroids are hormones that are synthesized in the central nervous system and are called steroids because they have a chemical structure similar to corticosteroids. Their functions are to protect, heal, and regenerate nerve tissue among other functions. For purposes of this primer, they heal and restore damaged nerve tissue to reduce chronic pain. Their clinical use is simple and relatively safe from side effects. Consequently, they are starting to emerge as a welcome addition to current pain care. The pain practitioner has multiple ways to incorporate neurosteroid therapy into the care of essentially every chronic or intractable pain case.

THE MAJOR NEUROSTEROIDS

A relatively small number of neurosteroids have been identified in the central nervous system (CNS). The major ones are pregnenolone, dehydroepiandrosterone (DHEA), progesterone, allopregnanolone, and androstenedione. The metabolic pattern is pictured here. DHEA metabolizes to estradiol and testosterone, and these well-known sex hormones may be called neurosteroids. Cortisol in not considered a neurosteroid. Androstenedione and allopregnanolone are neurosteroids but not available for clinical use, so they are not subjects in this "Primer." Neurosteroids are made in multiple CNS tissues including glial cells. They have their own receptors and relieve pain by interacting with the GABA and NMDA receptor complexes.

METABOLISM OF NEUROSTEROIDS

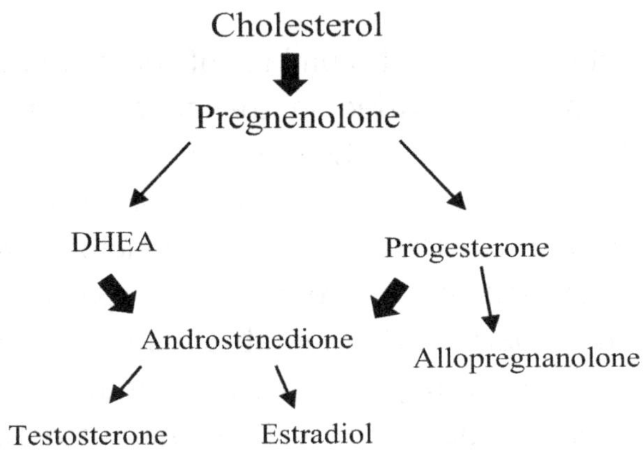

This diagram has skipped some steps in the entire NS metabolic pathway to show how the major neurosteroids are created. Estradiol and testosterone may or may not be considered neurosteroids. This handbook focuses only on pregnenolone, DHEA, and progesterone as they are clinically available for therapeutic use. Allopregnanolone and androstenedione are neurosteroids, but they are not available for medical purposes.

Critical Note: Neurosteroids in this primer refer only to DHEA, pregnenolone and progesterone.

FUNCTIONS OF NEUROSTEROIDS

Neurosteroids provide neuroprotection, healing of damaged tissues, and restoration (neuroregenesis) of damaged tissues. They reduce pain and neuroinflammation. They also naturally regulate stress, anxiety, cognition, and emotions. Neurosteroids relieve pain by direct interaction with the gamma amino butyric acid (GABA) and N-methyl-d-aspartate (NMDA) receptor complexes.

TABLE

Some NS Functions

Pain relief
Suppression of neuroinflammation
Neuroprotection
Neurorestoration (healing)
Neuroregenesis
Emotions
Cognition
Stress
Anxiety

Although neurosteroids are produced and function in the central nervous system (CNS), they are measurable in blood, urine, and spinal fluid.

USES OF NEUROSTEROIDS IN CHRONIC PAIN CARE

Neurosteroids have 4 basic uses in chronic pain care. As stated in the previous chapter, they are quite easy to administer and have few side effects. The Table below lists the 4 uses. Each use is described in detail in a later chapter.

TABLE

Uses of NS in Chronic Pain Care

1. Neurogenesis to repair tissues and decrease pain
2. Alternative to corticosteroids and anti-inflammatories
3. Enhancement of other pharmacologic agents
4. Potentiation of other treatments

SAFE AND EASY TO ADMINISTER

Neurosteroids are easy and safe to use in treating pain patients. They are taken orally. Pregnenolone and DHEA are widely available in multiple dosages. Deficiencies can be measured in blood. They seemingly have little adverse interaction when combined with other agents. Neurosteroids have proven to be almost side-effect free. Excess dosages dissipate rapidly and no severe complications or deaths are known to occur with them. The safety of neurosteroids makes it very practical to give a trial of a neurosteroid for about 20 to 30 days to see if a positive clinical reaction takes place. For example, a case of chronic fibromyalgia who takes an opioid and duloxetine can be given 50 mg of pregnenolone or DHEA for a 30-day trial with little concern for side-effects. The most common troublesome side effect is menstrual irregularity in premenopausal women who take a high dose of DHEA. Dosage may have to be restricted in premenopausal women.

HISTORY OF NEUROSTEROIDS

In the 1980's neuroscience researchers were immensely interested in the sex hormones, progesterone, estradiol, and testosterone and how they affected the central nervous system. The researchers determined that these hormones had an effect on the CNS because they identified specific receptors for these hormones in the CNS. In 1981, EE Balieu and his co-workers discovered dehydroepiandrosterone (DHEA) in rat brains. Two years later pregnenolone was discovered in the CNS. Researchers determined that these neurosteroids were derived from cortisol and metabolized to other neurosteroids. They didn't know their CNS functions, but they assumed they were behavior modulators. They determined that they had pain relieving effects on the gamma amino butyric acid (GABA) and N-methyl-D-aspartate receptors.

Beginning in 1990, a plethora of studies were done that demonstrated the profound power of

NS to heal CNS damage, restore tissues, and relieve pain.

A seminal study was done in which a combination of indomethacin, pregnenolone, and DHEA produced healing and restoration in rats with severed spinal cords. This study set a model and launched NS studies on the spine of laboratory animals.

Beginning in this century, clinical researchers began to determine if neurosteroids have a place in spinal trauma, stroke, and central pain. Blood levels of NS became available. A seminal study was done with US military personnel with chronic pain who returned from active duty in

the Middle East. Those veterans with chronic pain had very low levels of allopregnanolone which is a metabolite of progesterone. Other studies have shown that deficient levels of pregnenolone and other hormones are highly associated with chronic pain control.

The large number of laboratory animal studies have shown enough ability of neurosteroids to provide tissue healing and pain reduction to encourage clinical trials in humans. Open label administration of pregnenolone, DHEA, and medroxyprogesterone have been done by the author. At this point, neurosteroids are ready for routine clinical use and should become a critical component of chronic pain care.

<u>Étienne-Émile Baulieu</u>

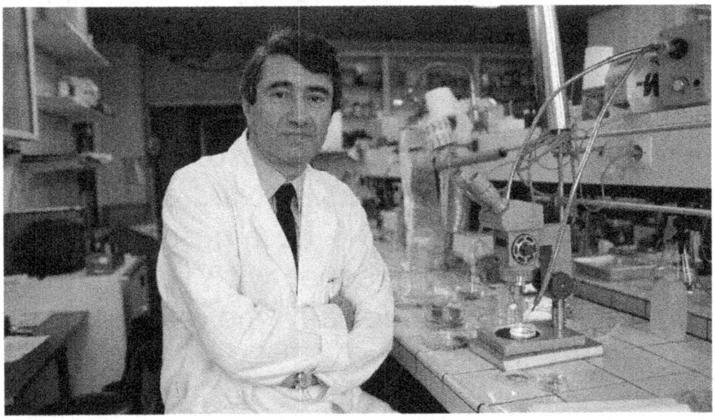

Etienne-Emile Baulieu discovered the first neurosteroid, dehydroepiandrosterone (DHEA) which is made in the central nervous system. (Year 1981)

PREGNENOLONE

Every pain practitioner should know some of the fascinating history of pregnenolone. It is also one of the most underutilized medicinals in chronic pain care.

Pregnenolone is derived from cholesterol, and it is the precursor of all the hormones produced in the adrenals or spinal cord. (See hormonal pathway in Chapter Three) During World War II, it was tested in factories and found to reduce fatigue and enhance energy and work productivity. The idea was to increase productivity during World War II. The author has observed many persons who take pregnenolone, and these performance enhancement traits are commonly recognized. Take a dose and you may feel energized. Also, in the 1940's, pregnenolone, along with implanted cortisone tablets, were the major treatment for rheumatoid arthritis. The dosage of pregnenolone required for pain relief was 400 to 600 mg a day. Pregnenolone use became almost extinct when prednisone was developed and marketed in the early 1950's. Prednisone seemed to be quicker acting and was easier to prescribe, but some observers at the time felt it was no more effective than pregnenolone. Big pharma marketing was alive and well in the early 1950's, so prednisone was successfully sold as a superior agent to pregnenolone.

In persons who cannot take a corticosteroid, the author recommends pregnenolone 200 mg in AM and PM. (Just like in 1945) To help determine if pregnenolone may assist chronic pain patients the author conducted two studies. In the first study 18 intractable pain patients with poor pain control were identified who had low serum pregnenolone

levels at the start of their pain treatment. Ninety days after entering treatment and after achieving some stabilization of pain, a repeat serum pregnenolone was determined. Serum pregnenolone rose to normal in 14 of the 18 (77.8%) and mean serum levels rose from 13.6 to 50.1 ng/ml ($p<.001$). This study indicates that good pain control requires normal blood levels of pregnenolone.

A second study involved 36 intractable pain patients who were enrolled in an ongoing intractable pain treatment program. All used opioids plus a variety of neuropathic and anti-inflammatory drugs. Chewable 10 mg pregnenolone tablets were offered to the 36 patients. They were allowed to chew as many as they needed or wanted to achieve better pain control and reduce other symptoms. At the end of 90 days, each participant was questioned as to whether pregnenolone helped their pain control and other symptoms including but not limited to energy, sleep, mental concentration, and less suffering or depression. Twenty-six of 36 (72.2%) reported improved pain relief and other symptoms. A total of 29 of 36 (80.6%) desired to continue pregnenolone after 90 days. There was about a 25% drop in opioid use. The dosage ranged widely from 10 to 120 mg a day. This study suggests that pregnenolone may improve pain control and other symptoms and showed some tendency to reduce opioid use.

One of the major attributes of pregnenolone is that it metabolizes to all other adrenal and gonadal hormones including progesterone and allopregnanolone. Both of these pregnenolone metabolites independently have potent pain relief properties. Arguably, pregnenolone should be given a 10-day trial in every chronic pain patient since it tends to minimize deficiencies of other hormones, enhance pain relief, and minimize opioids.

Interestingly, pregnenolone has never found a role in athletic enhancement but it clearly enhances mental and intellectual functions. This means it affects the glial cells, neurons, and receptors in the central nervous system. Pregnenolone is worthy of a 30-day trial in about every chronic pain patient.

TABLE

Quick Clinical Guide Pregnenolone Administration

- General supplement to prevent hormone deficiencies, 100 to 200 mg a day
- Alternative to corticosteroids, 200 mg in AM and PM

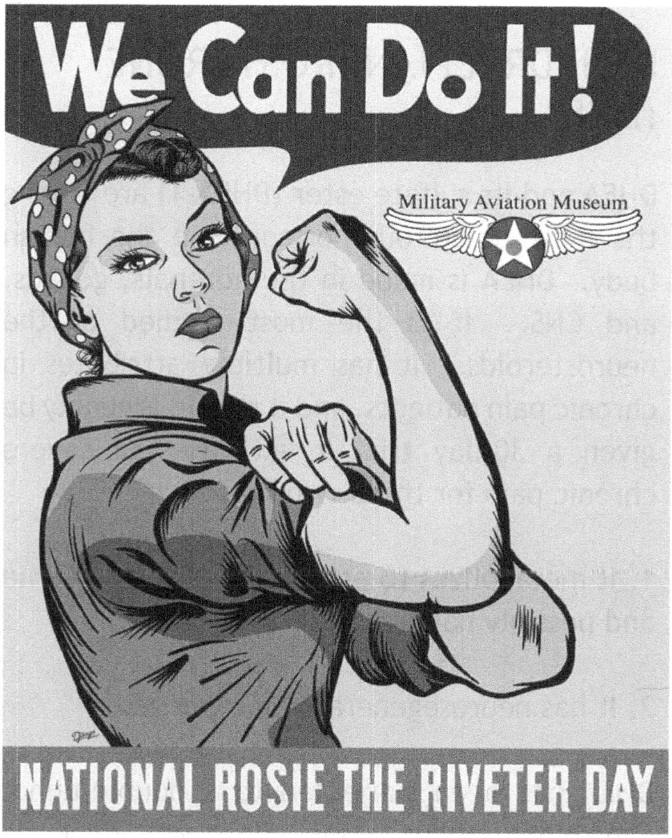

During World War II, pregnenolone was taken in factories to increase productivity. It was found to reduce fatigue and enhance energy.

DEHYDRPEPIANDROSTERONE (DHEA)

DHEA and its sulfate ester (DHEA-1) are among the most ubiquitous hormones in the human body. DHEA is made in the adrenals, gonads, and CNS. It is the most studied of the neurosteroids. It has multiple attributes in chronic pain patients, and it should arguably be given a 30-day trial in all cases of severe chronic pain for these two reasons:

1. It metabolizes to estradiol and testosterone and possibly nandrolone.

2. It has neuroregenerative properties

DHEA has been subjected to a double-blind, controlled study. This study was done on patients with systemic lupus erythematosus (SLE) who were severe enough to require corticosteroids and autoimmune agents. A daily dosage of 200 mg was found to reduce pain flares and reduce the chronic symptoms of baseline pain, lethargy, and depression.

DHEA may be found deficient in blood specimens taken from patients whose pain is poorly controlled. It should be replaced in this situation.

The attributes of DHEA include neuroregeneration and neuroprotection of both neurons and the glial cells that are responsible for constant central pain. DHEA also has anti-inflammatory properties and enhances the innate immune system. It has been shown to reduce interleukins, especially IL-10.

Although laboratories may differ, an adequate normal range is usually about 45 to 270 ug/dl. Some investigators recommend levels be kept above 200 ug/dl.

Given the documented benefits of DHEA, the author recommends a daily dose of DHEA be given a 30-day trial in almost all chronic pain patients. It can be used as a supplement to raise estradiol and testosterone, and/or used to enhance neuroregeneration and reduce pain. The starting dosage is 100 to 200 mg a day. This dosage can be increased to 400 mg a day given in divided dosages if given with pregnenolone as a corticosteroid substitute. The side effects reported with DHEA have been acne, loss of hair, and menstrual bleeding in premenopausal women. These side effects call for a reduced daily dosage.

TABLE

Quick Clinical Guide DHEA Administration

- Prevention of estradiol and testosterone deficiencies, 100 to 200 mg a day
- Promote neuroregeneration or corticosteroid alternative, 200 mg in AM and PM

TABLE

DHEA Attributes in Pain Treatment

- Reduce inflammation
- Enhances innate immune system
- Viral control
- Stimulates gamma aminobutyric acid and N-methyl-d-aspartate receptor for pain relief
- Decrease insulin resistance
- Neuroprotective and neuroregenerative effect on glial cells
- Increase testosterone and estradiol levels
- Alternative to corticosteroids

PROGESTERONE

Multiple basic science studies have established that progesterone has profound healing and neuroregeneration capabilities after a stroke or trauma to the brain or spinal cord. Its metabolite, allopregnanolone, was found to be low in studies of military men who had chronic pain and who returned from Middle East conflicts. These studies suggested that adequate pain relief has dependency on adequate serum levels of progesterone and allopregnanolone. Unfortunately, no studies were done on military veterans to determine which came first. Did low levels of allopregnanolone precede or follow the development of pain. Despite these studies in military persons with chronic pain, neither progesterone nor allopregnanolone has established a niche in chronic pain care.

Progesterone and its metabolite, allopregnanolone, are both produced in the central nervous system. Multiple studies show that these hormones are associated with neuroprotection, neuroregeneration, and myelin formation. (See attached references) Animal studies of spinal cord crush injuries show that progesterone accelerates the healing process. Enhanced recovery after stroke with progesterone is documented.

The author has used progesterone in two circumstances:

1. Low serum levels indicating a deficiency.

2. Patients who develop pain and other symptoms after a spinal tap, epidural injection, blood patch, or spine surgery. A dose of 100 to 200 mg a day for 7 to 10 days is used. It is combined with methylprednisolone in an attempt to minimize acute pain.

No systematic data has yet been collected, but preliminary observations by the author are that progesterone given with methylprednisolone may be effective in preventing adhesive arachnoiditis if symptoms develop after a medical procedure.

The only clinical study to demonstrate long-term pain relief that we can identify is a small open trial done by the author. Nine severe chronic pain patients were started on 10 mg of medroxyprogesterone. The dosage was raised to 20 to 40 mg a day over a period of 90 days. Six of the nine patients reduced their pain and reported an increase in energy, libido, and mental ability. Pain reduction was in the range of 20 to 30 percent. Daily opioid dosage was reduced in the 20 to 30 % range.

One of the reasons that progesterone has not yet been significantly used in pain care is that pregnenolone metabolizes to progesterone and allopregnanolone. Pregnenolone is an over-the-counter hormone that will raise progesterone and allopregnanolone blood levels. The pregnenolone supplement dosage is 100 to 200 mg a day.

Progesterone production may be reduced by both severe chronic pain and opioid administration. It should be replaced when found, by blood tests, to be deficient. Progesterone administration for ongoing chronic pain urgently needs trials as its effectiveness is likely underestimated.

TABLE

Quick Clinical Guide Progesterone Administration

- Replacement with low serum level, 100 mg a day
- Treatment of post-spinal tap, epidural injection, or surgery pain and neurologic symptoms, 100 to 200 mg for 10 days

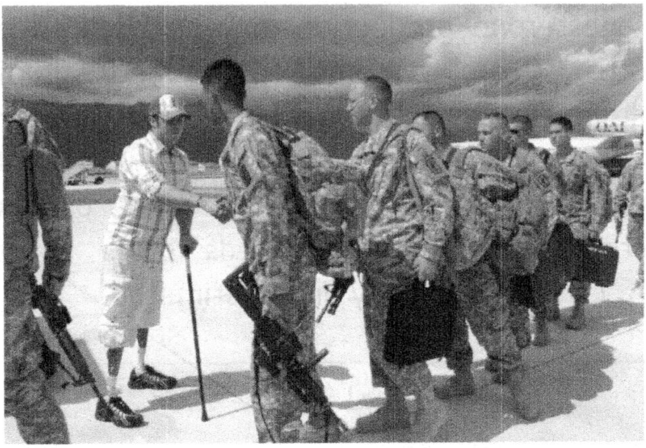

Soldiers returning from Middle East conflicts who had chronic pain were found to have low serum levels of allopregnanolone, a metabolite of pregnenolone and progesterone. It was undetermined if the low levels were the cause or result of the pain.

BLOOD TESTING FOR NEUROSTEROIDS

Blood levels of neurosteroids can now be easily accessed through essentially all community-based laboratories. The ability to determine blood levels of the critical neurosteroids is one reason that this primer could be written and that their use is a new practical addition to pain care. Blood samples can be taken any time of day and fasting is not necessary. The three critical neurosteroids for testing are pregnenolone, progesterone, and DHEA. Other hormones can be assessed in the same blood panel and include estradiol, testosterone, and cortisol.

To replenish deficient pregnenolone or DHEA blood levels, start oral administration at 50 mg a day and repeat the test in 30 days to determine if additional supplementation is needed.

It is important to note that both chronic pain and opioids may suppress NS. Both hormones appear to have a daily maximum output so the stress of chronic pain may exhaust or overwhelm the production of a neurosteroid. Simply put, determination of adequate blood levels of NS are usually necessary at some point in a person's chronic pain care.

TABLE

Replacement Dosages

Pregnenolone, DHEA, and progesterone start at 50 mg a day. Retest after 30 days.

THE NEUROGENIC USE OF NEUROSTEROIDS

A major, innate property of neurosteroids is to heal and regenerate damaged nerve tissues. Laboratory studies have shown the ability of neurosteroids to heal various tissues within the central nervous system including glial cells and axons. Healing and restoration of stroke and spinal cord damage has been well-documented (See References).

If a regenerative clinical purpose is intended, use both pregnenolone and DHEA together. Clinical situations would be applicable for such conditions as complex regional pain syndrome (CRPS), fibromyalgia, Ehlers-Danlos Syndrome, and neuropathies like pudendal neuropathy. Our considerable experience with neurosteroids and adhesive arachnoiditis is described in a later chapter.

The ongoing property of neurosteroids may be enhanced by a protein diet, amino acid-collagen supplement, and peptides.

The animal studies for this anabolic effect are well-documented. Multiple references are sited in this primer for pregnenolone, DHEA, and progesterone. Animal and human observations are well-matched. Neuroregeneration effects appear to target neural tissues, and glial cells responsible for controlling pain. The daily dosage for pregnenolone and DHEA are 100 to 200 mg twice a day. Progesterone's dosage is 100 to 200 mg a day. Progesterone's derivative medroxyprogesterone dosage is 20 to 30 mg a day.

To enhance the neuroregeneration effect I recommend simultaneous administration with peptides such as KPV, BPC-157, and ARA290 as well as amino acid/collagen supplements.

ALTERNATIVE TO CORTICOSTEROIDS AND ANTI-INFLAMMATORIES

Many chronic pain conditions have an inflammatory cause and/or propagator. Consequently, anti-inflammatory treatment may need to be long term or even lifetime. Long term administration of corticosteroids is problematic due to their multiple complications that include osteoporosis, hyperglycemia, obesity, and adrenal suppression. Anti-inflammatory agents also have long-term and short-term risks. These include gastrointestinal bleeding and glomerulonephritis. By and large neurosteroids are potent anti-inflammatory agents and avoid these potential complications. The major side effect with DHEA or progesterone and menstrual cycle side effects such as off-cycle bleeding.

Historically, pregnenolone, due to its anti-inflammatory properties, was used as the anti-inflammatory of choice for rheumatoid arthritis and systemic lupus prior to 1950 when prednisone was discovered. The daily dosage was usually between 400 to 600 mg a day. The advent of prednisone was hailed in the 1950's as superior to pregnenolone and easier to prescribe. Many physicians at that time disagreed, in that they believed pregnenolone was more effective than prednisone.

DHEA has not been used by itself as a corticosteroid alternative. It is given with pregnenolone. Together they have great ability as corticosteroid substitutions.

ENHANCEMENT OF OTHER PHARMACOLOGIC AGENTS

Neurosteroids have their own nociceptive or pain-relieving property. They have their own receptors in the central nervous system and interact at the GABA and NMDA receptor complexes to provide pain relief. Consequently, neurosteroids can be administered in low supplementary dosage and get some additional pain relief in patients who are taking opioids, neuropathic or anti-inflammatory agents. In a double-blind study of systemic lupus patients who were taking anti-inflammatory medication, pain was significantly reduced at a dosage of 200 mg a day. A small, open label study by me obtained a 25 to 46% pain reduction in intractable pain patients who used opioids as their main pain reliever. The dosage of medroxyprogesterone given was 10 mg a day for 30 days which resulted in a 20 to 30% reduction in opioid use.

Today many chronic pain patients have heard about neurosteroids and have on their own started supplementary pregnenolone and DHEA. Blood levels of progesterone and allopregnanolone are raised with use of oral pregnenolone. The starting dose can be as low as 10 to 20 mg a day. On our inquiry patients almost always report pain relief with these low pregnenolone dosages. The simplest way to initiate NS into chronic pain care is to start at a low supplementary dose for a 30-day trial. This is enough time to assess the benefit of neurosteroids.

<u>Dosages for Enhanced Pain Relief</u>

Pregnenolone, 100 to 200 mg a day
DHEA, 50 to 100 mg a day

NEUROSTEROIDS ARE NOT FOR ACUTE PAIN

Currently, neurosteroids have no systematic record of acute clinical use as does methylprednisolone or dexamethasone. At this time neurosteroids should be considered and used long term for chronic pain. Acute pain conditions such as post spinal puncture or herpes zoster infection should only be given one of the corticosteroids that have acute pain conditions as an indication. If the acute pain condition changes into a chronic condition a switch from corticoid treatment to neurosteroids should be considered. For example, the 6-day methylprednisolone (Medrol®) Dose Pak is commonly used in pain conditions. Neurosteroids can immediately follow the 6-day course if symptoms are still present.

CAUTION: NS are for chronic and not acute conditions. Acute pain requires a corticosteroid such as methylprednisolone.

POTENTIATION OF OTHER TREATMENTS

Described elsewhere in this primer is our treatment for adhesive arachnoiditis. It incorporates palmitoylethanolamide (PEA) into the combination of pregnenolone and DHEA. My belief is that neurosteroids potentiate or enhance some other medicinals used in pain care. Listed here are pain care medicinals that I have simultaneously given with neurosteroids. I have observed and believe they enhance the therapeutic effects of the medicinal.

A. Human Chorionic Gonadotropin (HCG)

This pituitary hormone has two biochemical units. One is a chain that consists of thyroid stimulating hormone (TSH), luteinizing hormone (LH), and follicle stimulating hormone (FSH). The other unit is purely a neuroregenerative neurohormone. Neurosteroids, when given with HCG, make a powerful neuroregeneration treatment.

B. Peptides

Several peptides have entered the commercial market and are being sold primarily for pain relief purposes. The most popular among chronic pain patients are KPV, BPC-157, and ARA290.

C. Oxytocin

Oxytocin is a neurohormone best known for its surge during childbirth for pain relief. It is now being used as an individual pain relief agent.

D. Nandrolone

Nandrolone is classified as an anabolic steroid, and its clinical indication is for wasting and debilitation. Traces of nandrolone can be found in spinal fluid so it may originate or be a metabolite of a neurosteroid such as DHEA. I have used nandrolone extensively in patients near end-of-life. Neurosteroids can be simultaneously given.

E. Palmitoylethanolamide (PEA)

PEA is a natural biologic molecule whose level rises in the body to reduce pain. It is produced in multiple tissues including glial cells. Its main biologic purpose is to heal, regenerate damaged tissues, and reduce pain. It appears to clinically be the best agent for central pain.

THE ARACHNOIDITIS TREATMENT

The major treatment of the inflammatory disease, adhesive arachnoiditis (AA) has been low dose methylprednisolone and ketorolac. Although an effective regimen for AA, the 2 agents carry a high burden of side-effects. Consequently, both patients and practitioners resist their use. To overcome the drawback of this treatment I have combined pregnenolone and DHEA with palmitoylethanolamide (PEA). PEA is a natural body analgesic that has healing, neurogenesis, and pain relief as its natural functions. It targets glial cells and neuroinflammation. It also promotes healing and neuroregeneration in the spinal cord. There are multiple double-blind studies showing it provides pain relief. Of keen interest is that it is increasingly being used successfully for central pain. The agents at this time appear clinically equal or superior to the standard, methylprednisolone and ketorolac. No systematic comparative evaluation has, however, been accomplished.

TABLE
Arachnoiditis Treatment

Pregnenolone, 200 mg twice a day
DHEA, 200 mg twice a day
PEA, 600 to 1200 mg twice a day

ALLOPREGNANOLONE - NO CLINICAL USE

Allopregnanolone is a neurosteroid and metabolite of progesterone. It primarily provides inhibition of electrical transmission in the central nervous system (CNS). In this role it acts as a neuropathic agent and has pain-relieving effects. Allopregnanolone, to my knowledge, has never been commercially available to medical practitioners. A synthetic formulation of allopregnanolone called brexanolone is approved by the US Food and Drug Administration for postpartum depression.

Allopregnanolone was found to be deficient in the blood of US Military veterans. This study shows that neurosteroids are naturally used for chronic pain and that adequate body levels are necessary for pain control. For unknown reasons allopregnanolone has not been clinically used and it is not available to practicing physicians.

FATE OF ANDROSTENEDIONE

In 1998 the baseball slugger Mark McGwire broke the record for a season by hitting 70 homeruns. Although this accomplishment was widely celebrated it was learned that he was taking the neurosteroid androstenedione when he got the record. At the time, it was legally sold over the counter as a dietary supplement. It became a popular sports enhancing agent and was known as "Andro." After the McGwire revelation androstenedione was banned by the US Food and Drug Administration. Sports agencies also banned its use and declared it was an anabolic steroid. It remains a banned substance today. Although there is no commercial androstenedione available today, it may be possible for physicians to obtain it as a special compounded agent. There are no clinical reports involving androstenedione and pain care.

Interestingly, androstenedione had become a popular supplement among pain patients in the years just prior to the McGwire affair. Patients claimed androstenedione potentiated opioids, reduced pain, and provided energy.

Unfortunately, no data was kept by me or others, as the ban on its medical use was unexpected.

Mark McGwire

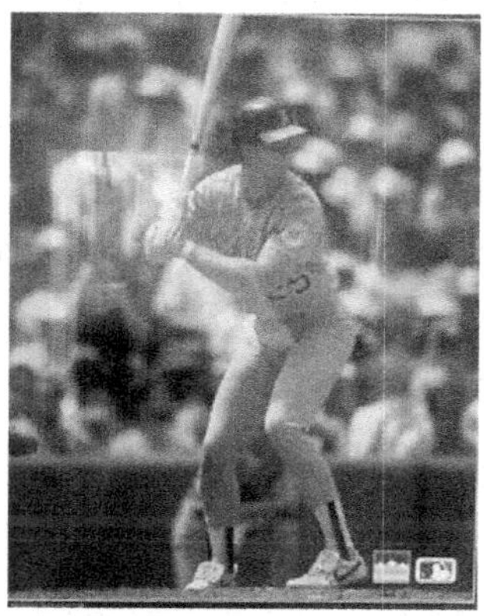

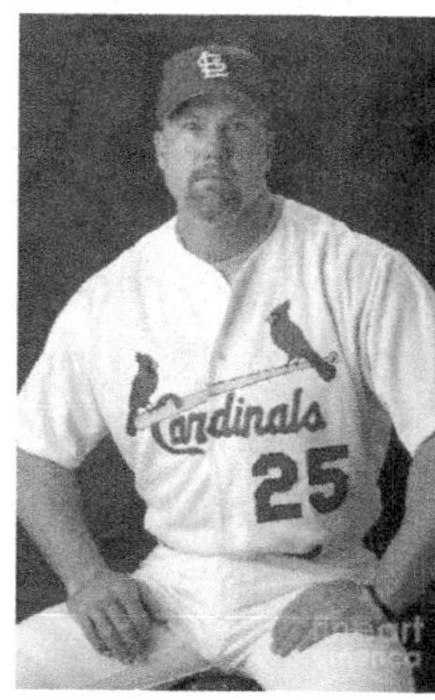

Androstenedione became a banned substance and was removed from the commercial market when it became known that baseball slugger Mark McGwire set a record of 70 homeruns in a season (1998).

SUMMARY

Neurosteroids are hormonal substances that are created in the brain and spinal cord. They have multiple effects on emotions, cognitive functions, and mood. They also have the functions of pain relief and neurogenesis. They relieve pain, in part, by stimulating the GABA and NMDA receptor complexes. Three neurosteroids, pregnenolone, DHEA, and progesterone, are accessible for chronic pain care. Neurosteroids can contribute to chronic pain care in 4 ways:

1. Restoration of damaged tissues
2. Enhance a patient's current pain regimen
3. Potentiate other medicinals and therapies
4. Alternative to corticosteroids and anti-inflammatories

In essence, enough animal and human data has been accumulated to recommend a role for neurosteroids in the care of almost every chronic pain patient.

REFERENCES

1. Aloisi A.M., Bonifazi M. Sex hormones, central nervous system and pain. *Hormones and Behavior*, 50, issue 1, 2006, 1-7.
2. Baulieu, EE, Robel P. Dehydroepiandrosterone (DHEA) and dehydroepiandrosterone sulfate (DHEAS) as neuroactive neurosteroids. *Proc Natl Acad Sci* 1998;95:4089-4091.
3. Bilello J, Tennant F. Patterns of chronic inflammation in extensively treated patients with arachnoiditis and chronic intractable pain. *Postgrad Med* 2016;92:1-5.
4. Blackburn-Munro G, Blackburn-Munro R. Pain in the brain: are hormones to blame? *Trends Endocrinol Metab* 2003 Jan;14(1):20-27.
5. Bracken MB, Shepard MJ, Thorpe K, et al. A randomized, controlled trial of methylprednisolone or naltrexone in the treatment of acute spinal cord injury: results of the Second National Acute Spinal Cord Injury Study. *N Engl J Med* 1990;322:1405-1411.
6. Breton JD, Veinante P, Uhi-Bronner S, et al. Oxytocin-induced antinociception in the spinal cord is mediated by a subpopulation of glutamatergic neurons in lamina-I-II which amplify GABAergic inhibition. *Mol Pain* 2008;4:19.
7. Ceccon M, Runbaugh G, Vincini S. Distinct effect of pregnenolone sulfate on NMDA receptor subtypes. *Neuropharm* 2001;40:491-500.
8. Chang DM, Chu SJ, Chen HC, et al. Dehydroepiandrosterone suppresses interleukin 10 synthesis in women with systemic lupus erythematosus. *Ann Rheum Dis* 63:1623-1620.

9. Compagnone NA, Mellon SH. Neurosteroids: biosynthesis and function of these novel neuromodulators. *Front Neuroendocrinol* 2000;21:1-56.
10. Coronel MF, Labomlorda F, Roig P, et al. Progesterone prevents allodynia after experimental spinal cord injury. J of Pain_2011;12:71-83.
11. Cutolo M. Estrogen metabolites: increasing evidence for their role in rheumatoid arthritis and systemic lupus erythematosus. *J Rheumatol* 2004;31:419-421.
12. Daniell HW. DHEA deficiency during consumption of sustained-action prescribed opioids: evidence for opioid-induced inhibition of adrenal androgen production. *J Pain* 2006;7:901-907.
13. Dawson-Basoa M, Gintzler AR. Estrogen and progesterone activate spinal kappa-opiate receptor analgesic mechanisms. *Pain* 1996;64:508-615.
14. Djeball M, Guo Q, Pertus EH, et al. The neurosteroids progesterone and allopregnanolone reduce cell death, gliosis, and functional deficits after traumatic brain injury in rate. *J Neurotrauma* 2005;22:106-118.
15. Engstrand B, Carlston K, Fellander-Tsai L, et al. Abnormal levels of serum dehydroepiandrosterone, estrone, and estradiol in men with rheumatoid arthritis: high correlation between serum estradiol and current degree of inflammation. *J Rheumatol* 2003;30:2338-2343.
16. Evrard HC, Balthazart J. Rapid regulation of pain by estrogen synthesized in spinal dorsal horn neurons. *J Neurosci* 2004;24:7225-7229.
17. Fischer L, Clementa JT, Tambeli CH. The protective role of testosterone in the development of temporomandibular joint pain. *J Pain* 2007;8:437-442.

18. Freeman H, Pincus G, Bachrach S, et al. Therapeutic efficacy of delta 5 pregnenolone in rheumatoid arthritis. *JAMA* 1950;143:338-344.
19. Gold J, High HA, Li Y, et sl. Safety and efficacy of nandrolone decanoate for treatment of wasting in patients with HIV infection. *AIDS* 1996 Jun;10(7):745-752.
20. Guth L, Zhang Z, Roberts E. Key role for pregnenolone in combination therapy that promotes recovery after spinal cord injury. *Proc Natl Acad Sci* 1994;91:12308-12312.
21. Harbuz MS, Perveen-Gill Z, Lightman SL, et al. A protective role for testosterone in adjuvant-induced arthritis. *Br J Rheumatol* 1995;34:1117-1122.
22. He J, Evans CO, Hoffman SW, et al. Progesterone and allopregnanolone reduce inflammatory cytokines after traumatic brain injury. *Exp Neuro* 2004;189:404-412.
23. Henderson E, Weinberg M, Wright WA. Pregnenolone. *J Clin Endo* 1950;10:455-474.
24. Joels M, DeKloet E. Control of neuronal excitability by corticosteroid hormones. *Trends Neurosci* 1992;15:25-30.
25. Jones KJ. Gonadal steroids and neuronal regeneration: a therapeutic role. *Adv Neurol* 1993;59:227-240.
26. Kilts JD, Tupler LA, Keefe FJ, et al. Neurosteroids and self-reported pain in veterans who served in the Military after September 11,2001. *Pain Med* 2010;10:1469-1476.
27. Lei ZM, Rao CV. Neural actions of luteinizing hormone and human chorionic gonadotropin. *Seminar Reprod Med* 2001;19:103-109.
28. McEwen BS, de Kloet ER, Rostene W. Adrenal steroid

receptors and action in the central nervous system. *Physio Rev* 1986;66:1121-1188.

29. McGavack TH, Chevalley J, Weissberg 1. The use Delta 5 pregnenolone in various clinical disorders. *J Clin Endocrinol* 1951;11(6):559-577.
30. Mensah-Nyagan A.G., Meyer L., Schaeffer V., et al. Evidence for a key role of steroids in the modulation of pain. *Psychoneuroendocrinology*, Volume 34, Issue SUPPL. 1, 2009, S169-S177.
31. Morlin R, Young J, Corpechot C, et al. Neurosteroids: pregnenolone in human sciatic nerves. *Proc Natl Acad Sci* 1992;98:6790-793.
32. Naylor JC, Kilts JD, Szabo ST, et al. Allopregnanolone levels with self-reported pain symptoms in U.S. Iraq and Afghanistan-Era veterans: Implications for biomarkers and therapeutics. *Pain Med* 2016;17:25-32.
33. Patil AA, Nagaraj MP. The effect of human chorionic gonadotropin (HCG) on functional recovery of spinal cord sectioned rats. *ACTA Neurochir* 1983;69:205-218.
34. Patill AA. The effect of human chorionic gonadotropin (HCG on restoration of the spinal cord. *Int Surg* 1990;75:54-57.
35. Pednekar J, Mulgaonker VK. Role of testosterone on pain threshold in rats. Indian *J Physiol Pharm*acol 1995;39:423-424.
36. Pincus G, Hoagland H. Effects of administered pregnenolone on fatiguing psychomotor performance. *Aviation Med* 1944;April:98-115.
37. Pincus G, Hoagland H. Effects on industrial production of the administration of delta 5 pregnenolone to factory workers. *I Psychosomatic Med* 1945;7:342-346.

38. Rash JA, Aguirre-Camacho A, Campbell TS. Oxytocin administration on acute cold pressor pain: a placebo-controlled, double-blind, within-subjects crossover trial. *Psychosom* Med 2014;76:422-429.
39. Reddy DS. Neurosteroids: endogenous role in the human brain and therapeutic potentials. *Prog Brain Res* 2010;186:13-137.
40. Roglio I, Bianchi R, Gotti S, et al. Neuroprotective effects of dehydroprogesterone and progesterone in an experimental model of nerve crush injury. *Neurosci* 2008 Aug 26;155(3):673-685.
41. Schverer M, Lanfumey L, Baulieu EE, et al. Neurosteroids: non-genomic pathways in neuroplasticity and involvement in neurological diseases. *Pharm & Ther* 2018 http://doi.org/10.1016/j.pharmthera.20.06.011.
42. Shealy CN. A review of dehydroepiandrosterone (DHEA). *Integ Physiol Behav* Sci 1995;30:308-313.
43. Shen W, Mennerick S, Covey DF, et al. Pregnenolone sulfate modulates inhibitory synaptic transmission by enhancing $GABA_a$ receptor desensitization. *J Neuroscience* 2000;20:3571-3579.
44. Tennant F. The physiologic effects of pain on the endocrine system. *Pain Ther* 2013 Dec;2(2):75-86.
45. Tennant F. Hormone abnormalities in severe, chronic pain patients who fail standard treatment. *Postgrad Med* 2015;127:1-4.
46. Tennant F. Clinical trial of progesterone for intractable, central pain. *Presented at Amer Acad Pain Med*, Palm Springs, CA 2012.
47. Tennant F. Human chorionic gonadotropin in pain treatment. *Prac Pain Manag* 2009;9:44-46.
48. Vallee M, Mayo W, Le Moal M. Role of pregnenolone, dehydroepiandrosterone and their sulfate esters on

learning and memory in cognitive aging. *Brain Res Brain Res Rev* 2001 ;37(1-3):301-12.

49. Webster KM, Wright DK, Sun M, et al. Progesterone treatment reduces neuroinflammation, oxidative stress and brain damage and improves long-term outcomes in a rat model of repeated mild traumatic brain injury. *J Neuroinflammation* 2015 Dec 18;12-238.

INDEX

OTHER BOOKS BY FOREST TENNANT

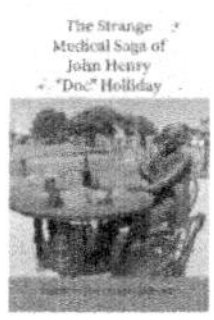

The Strange Medical Saga of "John Henry

ISBN: 9781955934275
LOC: 2023913628

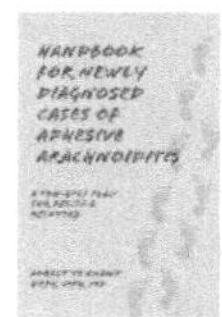

Handbook For Newly Diagnosed Cases of Adhesive Arachnoiditis

ISBN: 9781955934244
LOC: 2023908116

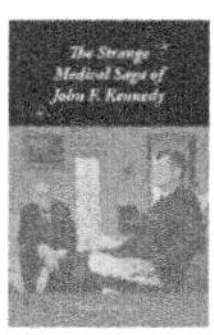

The Strange Medical Saga of JFK

ISBN: 9781955934213
LOC: 2023903440

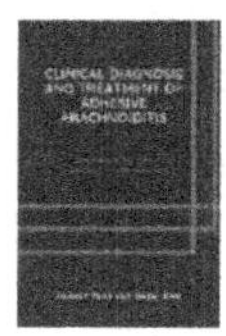

Clinical Diagnosis and Treatment of Adhesive Arachnoiditis

ISBN: 9781955934183
LOC: 2022907190

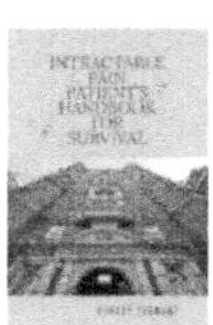

Intractable Pain Patients Handbook for Survival

ISBN: 9781955934121
LOC: 2021916464

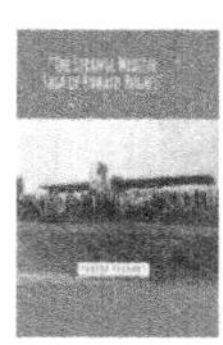

The Strange Medical Saga of Howard Hughes

ISBN: 9781955934091
LOC: 2021912855

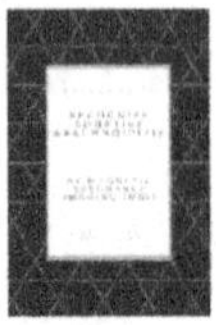

Handbook To Recognize Adhesive Arachnoiditis by Magnetic Resonance Imaging (MRI)

ISBN: 9781955934152
LOC: 2021925161

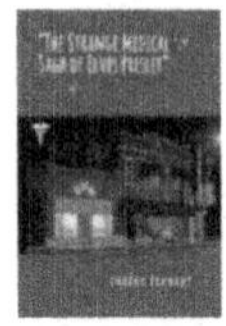

The Strange Medical Saga of Elvis

ISBN: 9781955934008
LOC: 2021911718

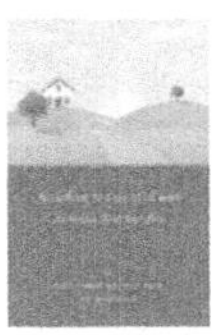

Handbook to Live Well with Adhesive Arachnoiditis

ISBN: 978195934060
LOC: 2021912718

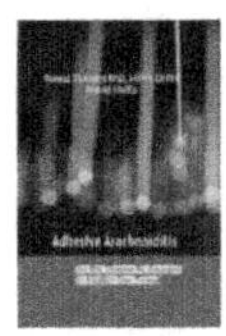

An Old Disease Re-Emerges in Modern Times

ISBN: 9781955934039
LOC: 2021912467

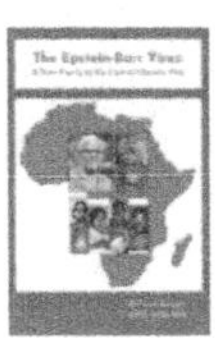

The Epstein-Barr Virus: A New Factor in the Care of Chronic Pain

ISBN: 9781955934428
LOC: 2024919179

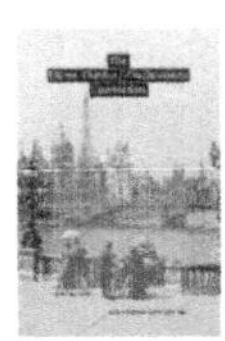

The Ehlers-Danlos / Arachnoiditis Connection

ISBN: 9781955934381
LOC: 2024911409

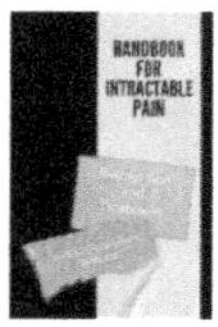

Handbook for Intractable Pain

ISBN: 9781955934329
LOC: 2023921074

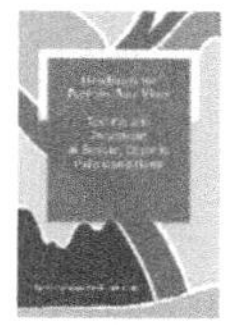

Handbook for Epstein-Barr Virus

ISBN: 9781955934459
LOC: 20249226413

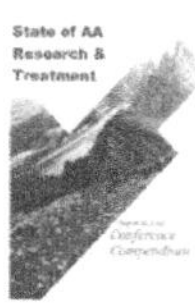

State of AA Research & Treatment Conference 2025

ISBN: 9781955934503
LOC: 2025918282

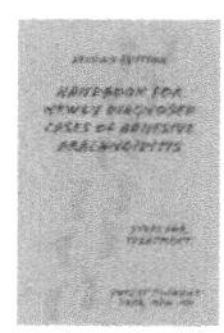

Second Edition Handbook For Newly Diagnosed Cases of Adhesive Arachnoiditis

ISBN: 9781955934480
LOC: 2025912299

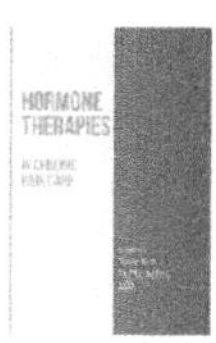

Hormone Therapies In Chronic Pain Care

ISBN:9781955934510
LOC:2026903164

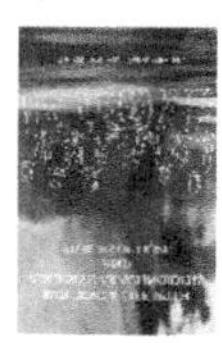

Building a Life With Adhesive Arachnoiditis And Stories Of Hope

ISBN: 9781955934466
LOC: 2026912281

Made in the USA
Monee, IL
16 September 2026

63296732R00036